Table Of Contents

Chapter 1: Health and Wellness

Importance of Regular Exercise

Regular exercise is crucial for maintaining good health and well-being, especially as we age. As we get older, our bodies tend to lose muscle mass and bone density, which can lead to a variety of health issues such as osteoporosis and muscle weakness. Engaging in regular physical activity can help combat these issues and improve overall strength and mobility.

Exercise is also important for maintaining a healthy weight and reducing the risk of chronic diseases such as heart disease, diabetes, and hypertension. By incorporating regular exercise into your routine, you can help lower your risk of developing these conditions and improve your overall quality of life. Additionally, exercise can help improve your mental health by reducing stress, anxiety, and depression.

Incorporating regular exercise into your daily routine doesn't have to be complicated or time-consuming. Simple activities such as walking, swimming, or gardening can provide numerous health benefits and help you stay active and independent as you age. It's important to find activities that you enjoy and that are suitable for your fitness level to ensure that you stick with them long-term.

In addition to the physical benefits, regular exercise can also help improve your cognitive function and reduce the risk of cognitive decline and dementia. Studies have shown that staying physically active can help improve memory, focus, and overall brain health. By making exercise a priority in your daily life, you can help maintain your cognitive function and stay sharp as you age.

Overall, regular exercise is essential for maintaining good health and well-being as a senior citizen. By staying active and incorporating physical activity into your daily routine, you can enjoy numerous benefits such as improved strength, mobility, and mental health. Remember to consult with your healthcare provider before starting a new exercise routine to ensure that it is safe and appropriate for your individual needs.

Tips for Healthy Eating

As we age, it becomes increasingly important to pay attention to our diet in order to maintain good health and vitality. In this subchapter, we will explore some tips for healthy eating that are specifically tailored to the needs of senior citizens. By following these guidelines, you can improve your overall well-being and reduce the risk of developing chronic diseases.

1. Focus on nutrient-dense foods: As we age, our bodies require fewer calories but more nutrients. It is important to choose foods that are rich in vitamins, minerals, and antioxidants. Include plenty of fruits, vegetables, whole grains, lean proteins, and healthy fats in your diet to ensure that you are getting all the essential nutrients your body needs.

2. Stay hydrated: Dehydration is a common problem among seniors and can lead to various health issues, such as urinary tract infections and constipation. Make sure to drink plenty of water throughout the day and include hydrating foods like fruits and vegetables in your diet. Avoid excessive consumption of caffeinated beverages and alcohol, as they can contribute to dehydration.

3. Practice portion control: As our metabolism slows down with age, it is important to be mindful of portion sizes to prevent weight gain. Use smaller plates and bowls to help control portion sizes and avoid overeating. Listen to your body's hunger and fullness cues, and stop eating when you feel satisfied, rather than when your plate is empty.

4. Limit processed foods and added sugars: Processed foods are often high in unhealthy fats, sodium, and added sugars, which can contribute to inflammation, weight gain, and chronic diseases. Opt for whole, unprocessed foods whenever possible and limit your intake of sugary snacks, desserts, and beverages. Choose natural sweeteners like honey or maple syrup instead of refined sugar.

5. Be mindful of special dietary needs: As we age, our bodies may become more sensitive to certain foods or nutrients. If you have any specific health conditions, such as diabetes, high blood pressure, or food allergies, work with a healthcare provider or registered dietitian to create a meal plan that meets your individual needs. Pay attention to how your body responds to different foods and make adjustments

as needed to support your overall health and well-being. By following these tips for healthy eating, you can nourish your body, boost your energy levels, and enjoy a higher quality of life as a senior citizen. Remember that small changes can lead to big improvements in your health, so start incorporating these guidelines into your daily routine today.

Understanding Common Health Conditions

As we age, it is important for senior citizens to be aware of common health conditions that can affect their well-being. By understanding these conditions, individuals can take proactive steps to prevent and manage them effectively. In this chapter, we will explore some of the most common health conditions that senior citizens may encounter as they age.

One common health condition that affects many senior citizens is arthritis. Arthritis is a condition that causes inflammation and stiffness in the joints, leading to pain and reduced mobility. There are several different types of arthritis, including osteoarthritis and rheumatoid arthritis. By staying active, maintaining a healthy weight, and following a balanced diet, individuals can help manage the symptoms of arthritis and improve their quality of life.

Another common health condition that senior citizens should be aware of is high blood pressure. High blood pressure, also known as hypertension, can increase the risk of heart disease, stroke, and other serious health problems. To keep blood pressure in check, individuals should monitor their blood pressure regularly, follow a low-sodium diet, and engage in regular physical activity. Medication may also be prescribed by a healthcare provider to help manage high blood pressure.

Cognitive decline is another health condition that can affect senior citizens, with Alzheimer's disease being one of the most common forms of dementia. As individuals age, they may experience memory loss, confusion, and difficulty with daily tasks. To help maintain cognitive function, it is important to stay mentally and socially active, engage in regular exercise, and eat a healthy diet rich in brain-boosting nutrients.

Diabetes is a chronic health condition that affects the body's ability to regulate blood sugar levels. For senior citizens, managing diabetes is crucial to prevent complications such as heart disease, kidney disease, and nerve damage. By monitoring blood sugar levels, following a healthy diet, and taking prescribed medications, individuals can effectively manage diabetes and live a full and active life.

In conclusion, understanding common health conditions is essential for senior citizens to maintain their well-being and quality of life as they age. By staying informed and taking proactive steps to prevent and manage these conditions, individuals can enjoy a healthy and fulfilling retirement. Remember, it is never too late to make positive changes to improve your health and well-being.

Chapter 2: Financial Planning

Managing Retirement Savings

Managing retirement savings is a crucial aspect of ensuring financial security in your golden years. As a senior citizen, it is important to carefully plan and monitor your retirement funds to make sure they last throughout your retirement. There are several key strategies to consider when managing your retirement savings to maximize your financial well-being.

One important step in managing retirement savings is to create a budget that outlines your expenses and income sources. By understanding your financial situation, you can make informed decisions about how to allocate your retirement funds. It is also important to regularly review and adjust your budget as needed to ensure that you are living within your means and saving for the future.

Another key aspect of managing retirement savings is to consider diversifying your investments. By spreading your investments across different asset classes, such as stocks, bonds, and real estate, you can reduce risk and potentially increase returns. It is important to work with a financial advisor to develop an investment strategy that aligns with your retirement goals and risk tolerance.

Monitoring your retirement savings on a regular basis is also essential for long-term financial security. By tracking your investments and reviewing your budget periodically, you can make adjustments as needed to stay on track with your retirement goals. It is important to stay informed about changes in the financial markets and consider how they may impact your retirement savings.

In conclusion, managing retirement savings is a critical aspect of financial planning for senior citizens. By creating a budget, diversifying investments, and monitoring your savings regularly, you can ensure that your retirement funds will last throughout your golden years. It is important to seek guidance from a financial advisor and stay informed about changes in the financial markets to make informed decisions about your retirement savings strategy.

Social Security Benefits

As a senior citizen, one of the most important benefits you may be entitled to is Social Security. Social Security benefits are designed to provide financial assistance to individuals who have reached retirement age, as well as to those who are disabled or have lost a spouse or parent. These benefits can help supplement your income and ensure that you have the financial security you need as you age. To qualify for Social Security benefits, you must have worked and paid into the Social Security system for a certain number of years. The amount of benefits you are entitled to will depend on your earnings history, as well as your age at the time you begin receiving benefits. It's important to understand how your benefits are calculated so that you can make informed decisions about when to start receiving them.

In addition to retirement benefits, Social Security also provides disability benefits for individuals who are unable to work due to a physical or mental impairment. These benefits can be a lifeline for those who are no longer able to support themselves through work. If you believe you may be eligible for disability benefits, it's important to apply as soon as possible to ensure that you receive the financial assistance you need.

Social Security benefits can also be available to surviving spouses and children of deceased workers. These benefits can help provide financial support to families who have lost a primary wage earner. If you are a surviving spouse or child, it's important to understand your rights and how to apply for these benefits.

Overall, Social Security benefits are a crucial source of financial support for many seniors. By understanding how these benefits work and what you may be entitled to, you can ensure that you receive the assistance you need to live comfortably in your retirement years. Be sure to stay informed about any changes to the Social Security system and how they may affect your benefits.

Estate Planning

Estate planning is a crucial aspect of preparing for the future, especially for senior citizens. It involves making decisions about how your assets will be distributed after your passing, as well as appointing a trusted individual to handle your affairs if you become incapacitated. By taking the time to create an estate plan, you can ensure that your wishes are carried out and that your loved ones are taken care of.

One of the key components of estate planning is creating a will. A will is a legal document that outlines how you want your assets to be distributed after your death. It allows you to specify who will inherit your property, money, and other possessions, as well as who will be responsible for carrying out your wishes. Without a will, your assets may be divided according to state laws, which may not align with your desires.

In addition to creating a will, it is important to consider other aspects of estate planning, such as setting up a trust. A trust is a legal arrangement that allows a third party, known as a trustee, to hold assets on behalf of a beneficiary. By establishing a trust, you can provide for the ongoing management and distribution of your assets, while also potentially reducing estate taxes and avoiding probate. Another important aspect of estate planning is appointing a power of attorney. A power of attorney is a legal document that grants someone the authority to make financial and medical decisions on your behalf if you are unable to do so. By selecting a trusted individual to act as your power of attorney, you can ensure that your affairs are handled in accordance with your wishes.

Overall, estate planning is a crucial step in preparing for the future and ensuring that your wishes are carried out. By creating a will, setting up a trust, and appointing a power of attorney, you can protect your assets, provide for your loved ones, and have peace of mind knowing that your affairs are in order. It is never too early to start estate planning, and it is essential for every senior citizen to consider their options and take action to secure their legacy.

Chapter 3: Technology and Social Media

Staying Safe Online

In today's digital age, staying safe online is more important than ever. As senior citizens, it's crucial to be aware of the potential risks and take steps to protect yourself while using the internet. This subchapter will provide you with valuable information on how to stay safe online and avoid falling victim to scams or identity theft. One of the key things to remember when it comes to staying safe online is to never share your personal information with strangers. This includes your full name, address, phone number, and especially your social security number. Scammers often try to trick people into giving out this information in order to steal their identity or commit fraud. Be cautious when entering your personal information on websites and only do so if you trust the site and know it is secure. Another important step in staying safe online is to use strong and unique passwords for all of your online accounts. Avoid using easily guessed passwords such as "123456" or "password" and instead create complex passwords with a mix of letters, numbers, and special characters. It's also a good idea to change your passwords regularly and enable two-factor authentication whenever possible to add an extra layer of security to your accounts.

When browsing the internet, be wary of unsolicited emails, messages, or pop-up ads that may contain malicious links or attachments. These could be phishing attempts designed to trick you into revealing your personal information or downloading malware onto your device. Always verify the source of the message before clicking on any links or opening any attachments, and never provide sensitive information in response to an unsolicited request.

Lastly, consider using security software on your devices to help protect yourself from online threats. Antivirus programs, firewalls, and ad blockers can all help to keep your personal information safe while browsing the web. By taking these simple precautions and staying informed about the latest online threats, you can enjoy the benefits of the internet while keeping yourself safe from harm.

Using Social Media to Stay Connected

In today's digital age, social media has become an essential tool for staying connected with friends and family. As a senior citizen, you may feel intimidated by the idea of using social media, but it can actually be a fun and easy way to keep in touch with loved ones. This subchapter will provide you with valuable information on how to use social media to stay connected and engaged in the digital world.

One of the most popular social media platforms for seniors is Facebook. This platform allows you to connect with friends and family, share photos and updates, and join groups with shared interests. Creating a Facebook account is simple and free, and once you're set up, you can start connecting with people right away. You can also use Facebook to stay up to date on news and events in your community.

Another great way to stay connected through social media is by using video calling apps like Skype or FaceTime. These apps allow you to have face-to-face conversations with friends and family, even if they're far away. Video calling can help you feel more connected and reduce feelings of isolation, especially if you live alone. It's also a great way to see your loved ones' faces and share special moments with them.

Twitter is another social media platform that can help you stay connected with the world around you. On Twitter, you can follow your favorite celebrities, news outlets, and organizations to stay informed on current events and trends. You can also tweet your own thoughts and opinions, and engage with others in conversations. Twitter can be a great way to stay connected with the larger community and have your voice heard.

In conclusion, social media can be a valuable tool for staying connected and engaged as a senior citizen. Whether you're using Facebook to connect with friends and family, video calling apps to have face-to-face conversations, or Twitter to stay informed on current events, social media can help you feel more connected to the world around you. Don't be afraid to explore these platforms and see how they can enhance your social connections and overall well-being.

Helpful Apps for Seniors

As technology continues to advance, there are more and more apps available that can make life easier for seniors. In this subchapter, we will explore some helpful apps that can assist senior citizens in various aspects of their lives. These apps can help with everything from staying connected with loved ones to managing medications and staying active.

One of the most popular apps for seniors is Zoom, a video conferencing app that allows users to connect with family and friends from anywhere in the world. With Zoom, seniors can participate in virtual family gatherings, attend virtual doctor's appointments, and even join online exercise classes. This app is particularly useful for seniors who may be unable to travel or visit loved ones in person.

Another helpful app for seniors is Medisafe, a medication management app that helps users keep track of their medications and dosages. With Medisafe, seniors can set reminders for when to take their medications, track their medication history, and even receive alerts if they miss a dose. This app can help seniors stay on top of their health and ensure they are taking their medications as prescribed.

For seniors looking to stay active and maintain a healthy lifestyle, the Fitbit app is a great tool. This app can track steps, monitor heart rate, and even provide guided workouts and meditation sessions. Seniors can set fitness goals, track their progress, and stay motivated to stay active and healthy. The Fitbit app is a great way for seniors to stay on top of their physical health and wellness.

In addition to these apps, there are many others that can benefit seniors in different ways. From grocery delivery apps to transportation apps to mental health and mindfulness apps, there is something for everyone. By exploring and utilizing these helpful apps, seniors can stay connected, manage their health, and live their best lives. It's never too late to embrace technology and all the ways it can improve our lives as seniors.

Chapter 4: Travel and Leisure

Senior Discounts and Deals

As a senior citizen, you may be entitled to a variety of discounts and deals that can help you save money on everyday expenses. From dining out to shopping for groceries, there are many opportunities for seniors to take advantage of special offers and promotions. In this subchapter, we will explore some of the best senior discounts and deals available to help you make the most of your retirement years. One of the most common types of senior discounts is offered by restaurants and fast food chains. Many establishments offer discounted meals or special deals for seniors, making dining out more affordable for those on a fixed income. By presenting your AARP card or another form of identification, you can enjoy savings on your favorite meals at a variety of restaurants.

In addition to dining discounts, seniors can also save money on groceries and household items by taking advantage of senior discounts at supermarkets and retail stores. Many grocery stores offer special discount days for seniors, where you can save a percentage off your total purchase. By planning your shopping trips around these discount days, you can stretch your budget further and stock up on essentials for less.

When it comes to entertainment and leisure activities, seniors can also benefit from special discounts and deals. Many movie theaters, museums, and attractions offer discounted admission for seniors, making it easier to enjoy a day out without breaking the bank. By researching local attractions and venues that offer senior discounts, you can plan fun and affordable outings that won't strain your budget.

In conclusion, senior discounts and deals are a great way for seniors to save money and make the most of their retirement years. By taking advantage of discounts on dining, groceries, entertainment, and more, you can stretch your budget further and enjoy a higher quality of life. Be sure to research the discounts available in your area and take advantage of the savings opportunities that are available to you as a senior citizen.

Tips for Safe Travel

Traveling can be an exciting and rewarding experience for senior citizens, but it's important to take certain precautions to ensure a safe journey. Here are some tips for safe travel that every senior should know:

1. Plan ahead: Before embarking on your trip, make sure to do some research about your destination. Check the weather forecast, familiarize yourself with local customs and laws, and make a list of important contacts such as your embassy or consulate. It's also a good idea to share your itinerary with a friend or family member in case of emergencies.

2. Pack wisely: When packing for your trip, be sure to bring any necessary medications, a copy of your prescriptions, and a list of your medical conditions and allergies. It's also a good idea to pack a first aid kit, travel insurance information, and a list of emergency

contacts. Don't forget to pack comfortable clothing and shoes to ensure a pleasant journey.

3. Stay vigilant: While traveling, it's important to stay alert and aware of your surroundings. Keep an eye on your belongings at all times, be cautious of strangers, and avoid displaying valuables such as jewelry or large amounts of cash. If you're traveling alone, consider joining a tour group or using a reputable travel agency for added security.

4. Stay connected: Make sure to keep in touch with your loved ones while traveling. Consider purchasing an international phone plan or a portable Wi-Fi device to stay connected with friends and family back home. It's also a good idea to carry a charged cell phone with emergency contacts programmed in case of an unexpected situation.

5. Take care of yourself: Traveling can be exhausting, so make sure to take care of yourself during your journey. Stay hydrated, get plenty of rest, and take breaks when needed. If you have any mobility or health concerns, consider requesting assistance or accommodations in advance to ensure a smooth and enjoyable trip.

By following these tips for safe travel, senior citizens can enjoy their adventures with peace of mind and confidence. Remember to always prioritize your safety and well-being while exploring new destinations. Safe travels!

Exploring New Hobbies

As we age, it's important to stay active and engaged in order to maintain a healthy and fulfilling lifestyle. One way to do this is by exploring new hobbies. Whether you're looking to pick up a new skill or simply try something different, there are a wide variety of hobbies to choose from that can help keep your mind sharp and your spirits high.

One popular hobby among seniors is gardening. Not only is gardening a great way to get some exercise and fresh air, but it also allows you to connect with nature and see the fruits of your labor come to life. Whether you have a small balcony or a large backyard, there are plenty of options for creating a beautiful garden that you can enjoy year-round.

Another hobby to consider is painting or drawing. Many seniors find that expressing themselves through art can be a therapeutic and relaxing experience. Whether you're a beginner or an experienced artist, there are plenty of resources available to help you get started and improve your skills. Plus, you can create beautiful pieces of artwork to display in your home or give as gifts to loved ones.

If you're looking for a hobby that gets you moving, consider taking up a new form of exercise such as yoga or tai chi. These gentle forms of exercise can help improve your balance, flexibility, and overall well-being. Plus, they can be easily modified to fit your individual needs and abilities, making them a great option for seniors of all fitness levels.

Finally, don't be afraid to try something completely out of your comfort zone. Whether it's learning a new language, taking up a musical instrument, or trying your hand at cooking a new cuisine, exploring new hobbies can help you discover new passions and interests that you never knew you had. So go ahead, step out of your comfort zone and try something new – you never know what you might discover about yourself in the process.

Chapter 5: Home Safety and Maintenance

Preventing Falls

Preventing falls is an important aspect of maintaining good health and independence as we age. As we get older, our bodies may not be as strong or stable as they once were, making us more susceptible to accidents. However, there are steps that senior citizens can take to reduce their risk of falling and stay safe in their daily activities.

One of the most effective ways to prevent falls is to stay active and engaged in regular physical activity. Exercise helps to improve strength, balance, and flexibility, all of which are important for preventing falls. By incorporating activities such as walking, swimming, or tai chi into your routine, you can help maintain your physical health and reduce your risk of falling.

In addition to staying active, it is important for senior citizens to make their living environment safe and free of hazards. This can include removing clutter from walkways, installing grab bars in the bathroom, and ensuring that rugs are secure and do not pose a tripping hazard. By taking these simple steps, you can create a safer environment that reduces your risk of falling at home.

Another important aspect of fall prevention is to review your medications with your healthcare provider. Some medications can cause dizziness or lightheadedness, which can increase your risk of falling. By discussing your medications with your doctor and making any necessary adjustments, you can help reduce this risk and stay safe.

Overall, preventing falls is an important part of staying healthy and independent as a senior citizen. By staying active, creating a safe living environment, and reviewing your medications, you can significantly reduce your risk of falling and enjoy a more active and fulfilling lifestyle. Remember, it's never too late to take steps to prevent falls and protect your well-being.

Fire Safety Tips

Fire safety is a crucial aspect of ensuring the well-being of senior citizens in their homes. In this subchapter, we will explore some important fire safety tips that every senior should be aware of in order to prevent accidents and ensure their safety.

First and foremost, it is important to have working smoke detectors installed in your home. Smoke detectors are your first line of defense in case of a fire, as they can alert you to the presence of smoke and give you valuable time to evacuate safely. Make sure to test your smoke detectors regularly and replace the batteries at least once a year to ensure they are in working condition.

In addition to smoke detectors, it is important to have a fire extinguisher in your home. Keep the fire extinguisher in an easily accessible location, such as the kitchen or near the bedroom, and make sure you know how to use it properly. In case of a small fire, you can use the fire extinguisher to put it out before it spreads.

Another important fire safety tip is to have an escape plan in place. Make sure all doors and windows in your home are easily accessible and can be opened quickly in case of an emergency. Practice your escape plan with your family members or caregivers so that everyone knows what to do in case of a fire.

Finally, it is important to be cautious when using appliances and candles in your home. Make sure to turn off appliances when not in use and never leave candles unattended. Keep flammable items such as curtains, towels, and clothing away from heat sources to prevent accidental fires. By following these fire safety tips, you can help protect yourself and your home from the dangers of fire.

Home Maintenance Checklist

Home maintenance is an important aspect of senior living that often gets overlooked. As we age, it becomes even more crucial to stay on top of regular home maintenance tasks to ensure our safety and comfort. This Home Maintenance Checklist will help you stay organized and proactive in taking care of your living space.

First and foremost, it's essential to check your smoke detectors and carbon monoxide detectors regularly. These devices can save your life in the event of a fire or gas leak, so be sure to test them monthly and replace the batteries at least once a year. Additionally, make sure to have a fire extinguisher in your home and check that it is in good working condition.

Next, take a walk around your home and inspect for any potential safety hazards. Look for loose rugs or cords that could cause tripping, as well as any areas of the floor that may be uneven. Keep pathways clear of clutter and make sure there is adequate lighting in all rooms to prevent falls.

Another important task on your Home Maintenance Checklist is to check your plumbing and electrical systems. Look for any signs of leaks, such as water stains on walls or ceilings, and have them repaired promptly. Check that all electrical outlets and switches are working properly and have a professional inspect your wiring if you notice any flickering lights or other electrical issues.

Don't forget about the exterior of your home when it comes to maintenance. Inspect your roof for any missing or damaged shingles, and clean out your gutters to prevent water damage. Trim back any overgrown bushes or trees that may be encroaching on your home, and make sure your walkways and driveway are in good repair to prevent slips and falls.

By following this Home Maintenance Checklist, you can ensure that your living space remains safe and comfortable for years to come. Taking care of these tasks regularly will not only help prevent costly repairs down the line but will also give you peace of mind knowing that your home is in good condition. Remember, it's never too late to start prioritizing your home maintenance as a senior citizen.

Chapter 6: Mental Health and Wellbeing

Coping with Loneliness

Loneliness is a common experience for many seniors, especially those who may have lost a spouse or close friends. Coping with loneliness can be challenging, but there are strategies that can help you feel more connected and supported. In this subchapter, we will explore some tips and techniques for dealing with loneliness and finding ways to stay socially engaged.

One way to cope with loneliness is to stay active and engaged in activities that you enjoy. This can help you meet new people and build connections with others who share your interests. Consider joining a club or group that focuses on a hobby or activity you enjoy, such as gardening, painting, or reading. This can provide you with a sense of community and companionship that can help combat feelings of isolation.

Another way to cope with loneliness is to reach out to family and friends for support. Don't be afraid to ask for help or company when you need it. You may find that loved ones are more than willing to spend time with you and provide the companionship you need. Consider scheduling regular visits or phone calls with friends and family members to stay connected and maintain relationships that are important to you.

If you are feeling lonely, consider volunteering your time and skills to help others in need. Volunteering can provide you with a sense of purpose and fulfillment, as well as opportunities to meet new people and make a positive impact in your community. Look for local organizations or charities that could benefit from your time and expertise, and consider how you can contribute to their mission.

It's important to take care of your mental and emotional well-being while coping with loneliness. Consider seeking support from a therapist or counselor who can help you navigate your feelings and develop coping strategies. You may also find comfort in practicing mindfulness or meditation to help calm your mind and reduce feelings of loneliness. Remember that it's okay to seek help and support when you need it, and that there are resources available to help you cope with loneliness in healthy and productive ways.

In conclusion, coping with loneliness can be a challenging experience for many seniors, but there are strategies that can help you feel more connected and supported. By staying active and engaged in activities you enjoy, reaching out to loved ones for support, volunteering your time, and taking care of your mental and emotional well-being, you can combat feelings of loneliness and find ways to stay socially engaged. Remember that it's important to prioritize your own well-being and seek support when you need it.

Strategies for Stress Management

Stress is a common issue that many seniors face in their daily lives, but there are effective strategies that can help manage and reduce stress levels. In this subchapter, we will explore some key strategies for stress management that can help improve your overall well-being and quality of life.

One important strategy for managing stress is to practice relaxation techniques such as deep breathing, meditation, or yoga. These techniques can help calm your mind and body, reduce muscle tension, and promote feelings of relaxation and calmness. Taking a few minutes each day to practice these techniques can have a significant impact on your stress levels.

Another effective strategy for managing stress is to engage in regular physical activity. Exercise has been shown to reduce stress levels, improve mood, and boost overall well-being. Whether it's going for a walk, taking a dance class, or practicing tai chi, finding an activity that you enjoy and can do regularly can help alleviate stress and improve your mental and physical health.

In addition to relaxation techniques and physical activity, maintaining a healthy lifestyle can also help reduce stress. Eating a balanced diet, getting enough sleep, and staying hydrated are all important factors in managing stress levels. Avoiding excessive alcohol consumption, smoking, and caffeine can also help reduce stress and improve your overall health.

Finally, seeking support from friends, family, or a counselor can also be beneficial in managing stress. Talking to someone about your feelings and concerns can help you feel more supported and less alone in dealing with stress. Remember, it's okay to ask for help when you need it, and seeking support from others can be an important part of managing stress effectively. By incorporating these strategies into your daily routine, you can better manage stress and improve your overall well-being as a senior citizen.

Importance of Mental Health Check-ups

As we age, it is important to prioritize our mental health just as much as our physical health. Mental health check-ups are crucial for maintaining overall well-being and ensuring a high quality of life in our senior years. In this subchapter, we will explore the importance of mental health check-ups for senior citizens and why they should be a regular part of our healthcare routine.

First and foremost, mental health check-ups allow seniors to address any potential issues or concerns early on. Just like with physical health, early detection and intervention can make a significant difference in the outcome of mental health conditions. By regularly checking in with a mental health professional, seniors can receive the support and resources they need to manage any challenges they may be facing.

Additionally, mental health check-ups can help seniors stay socially connected and engaged with their communities. As we age, it is common for social isolation to become a problem, which can have negative effects on our mental well-being. Regular check-ups can provide seniors with opportunities to discuss their feelings, connect with others, and seek out resources for staying engaged and active. Furthermore, mental health check-ups can help seniors cope with the many changes and challenges that come with aging. From adjusting to retirement to dealing with health issues, seniors may face a variety of stressors that can impact their mental health. By regularly checking in with a mental health professional, seniors can develop coping strategies and receive support for managing these life transitions.

In conclusion, mental health check-ups are an essential part of maintaining overall well-being in our senior years. By prioritizing our mental health and seeking out regular check-ups, we can address any issues early on, stay socially connected, and cope with the challenges of aging. Remember, it is never too late to prioritize your mental health and take steps towards a happier and healthier future.

Chapter 7: Legal Rights and Advocacy

Understanding Medicare and Medicaid

Medicare and Medicaid are two important government programs that provide health insurance coverage for millions of Americans, including senior citizens. In this subchapter, we will explore the differences between these two programs and how they can benefit you as a senior citizen.

Medicare is a federal health insurance program for people aged 65 and older, as well as for certain younger individuals with disabilities. It is divided into several parts, including Part A (hospital insurance), Part B (medical insurance), Part C (Medicare Advantage plans), and Part D (prescription drug coverage). Medicare helps cover a wide range of medical services, including hospital stays, doctor visits, and prescription medications.

Medicaid, on the other hand, is a joint federal and state program that provides health insurance coverage to low-income individuals, including senior citizens with limited financial resources. Medicaid covers a broader range of services than Medicare, including long-term care, nursing home care, and home health services. Eligibility for Medicaid is based on income and asset limits set by each state.

It is important for senior citizens to understand the differences between Medicare and Medicaid, as well as how to enroll in these programs. Medicare enrollment usually begins three months before your 65th birthday and ends three months after. Medicaid enrollment can be done at any time, but eligibility requirements vary by state. If you are eligible for both Medicare and Medicaid, you may be able to receive benefits from both programs to help cover your healthcare costs.

In conclusion, Medicare and Medicaid are vital programs that provide health insurance coverage to millions of Americans, including senior citizens. By understanding the differences between these two programs and how to enroll in them, you can ensure that you have access to the healthcare services you need as you age. Whether you are eligible for Medicare, Medicaid, or both, it is important to take advantage of these programs to protect your health and financial well-being in your golden years.

Power of Attorney and Living Wills

As we age, it's important to plan for the future and make decisions about our healthcare and finances in case we are unable to do so ourselves. One way to ensure your wishes are carried out is by establishing a Power of Attorney. A Power of Attorney is a legal document that grants someone the authority to make decisions on your behalf if you become incapacitated. This person, known as your agent or attorney-in-fact, can make decisions about your healthcare, finances, and other important matters. It's important to choose someone you trust to act in your best interests.

Another important document to consider is a Living Will. A Living Will, also known as an advance directive, allows you to specify your wishes for medical care in the event you are unable to communicate them yourself. This document outlines the type of medical treatment you want or don't want, such as life-sustaining measures or organ donation. By creating a Living Will, you can ensure your healthcare providers and loved ones know your preferences and can make decisions that align with your wishes.

Having a Power of Attorney and Living Will in place can provide peace of mind for both you and your loved ones. These documents help ensure your wishes are honored and can prevent disputes or confusion during times of crisis. It's important to review and update these documents regularly to reflect any changes in your health or personal circumstances. By taking proactive steps to plan for the future, you can ease the burden on your loved ones and ensure your wishes are respected.

In addition to a Power of Attorney and Living Will, it's also important to discuss your end-of-life preferences with your loved ones. Having open and honest conversations about your wishes for medical care, funeral arrangements, and other important decisions can help your family members understand and respect your choices. By planning ahead and communicating your desires, you can help alleviate stress and uncertainty for your loved ones during difficult times.

In conclusion, creating a Power of Attorney and Living Will are essential steps in planning for the future and ensuring your wishes are carried out. These documents provide legal protection and clarity for both you and your loved ones. By taking the time to establish these important documents and have important conversations with your family, you can have peace of mind knowing your wishes will be honored and your loved ones will be supported during challenging times.

Resources for Legal Assistance

When facing legal issues, it is crucial for senior citizens to have access to the proper resources for legal assistance. Whether you are dealing with estate planning, elder abuse, or any other legal matter, having the right support can make all the difference. In this subchapter, we will explore some key resources that can help seniors navigate the legal system and protect their rights.

One valuable resource for legal assistance is the Legal Aid Society, which provides free or low-cost legal services to individuals who cannot afford traditional legal representation. This organization has offices across the country and can help seniors with a wide range of legal issues, including housing, consumer rights, and family law. By contacting the Legal Aid Society, seniors can connect with experienced attorneys who can provide guidance and representation.

Another important resource for seniors seeking legal assistance is the National Academy of Elder Law Attorneys (NAELA). This organization is dedicated to serving the legal needs of older adults and individuals with disabilities. NAELA members are well-versed in elder law issues, such as Medicaid planning, long-term care planning, and guardianship. By finding a NAELA attorney in their area, seniors can ensure they are receiving expert legal advice tailored to their specific needs.

In addition to these organizations, many local bar associations offer pro bono legal services for seniors. These programs connect seniors with volunteer attorneys who can provide legal advice and representation at no cost. By reaching out to their local bar association, seniors can access valuable legal assistance without breaking the bank. This can be especially helpful for seniors on a fixed income who may not be able to afford expensive legal fees.

Lastly, seniors can also turn to their state's department of aging for legal assistance. Many state agencies offer legal aid programs specifically for seniors, which can provide guidance on a variety of legal issues, from Medicare and Social Security benefits to elder abuse and neglect. By contacting their state's department of aging, seniors can access resources and support to help them navigate the complex legal system and protect their rights.

In conclusion, having access to the right resources for legal assistance is essential for senior citizens facing legal challenges. By seeking out organizations like the Legal Aid Society, NAELA, local bar associations, and state departments of aging, seniors can ensure they receive the legal support they need to protect their rights and interests. By utilizing these resources, seniors can navigate the legal system with confidence and peace of mind.

Chapter 8: Social Activities and Community Engagement

Joining Senior Centers and Clubs

Senior centers and clubs are wonderful places for older adults to socialize, stay active, and engage in various activities. These centers provide a welcoming environment where seniors can make new friends, participate in exercise classes, learn new skills, and enjoy stimulating discussions. Joining a senior center or club can greatly enhance your quality of life as you age.

One of the key benefits of joining a senior center or club is the opportunity to meet like-minded individuals who share your interests and experiences. These centers often host a wide range of activities and events, from book clubs and art classes to fitness programs and group outings. By joining a senior center or club, you can connect with others who are going through similar life stages and build lasting friendships.

In addition to socializing and participating in activities, senior centers and clubs also offer valuable resources and support services for older adults. Many centers provide access to health and wellness programs, educational workshops, and information on community resources. By becoming a member of a senior center or club, you can gain access to a wealth of information and support that can help you navigate the challenges of aging.

Joining a senior center or club can also have a positive impact on your mental and emotional well-being. Research has shown that social isolation and loneliness can have negative effects on health, including an increased risk of depression and cognitive decline. By joining a senior center or club, you can combat feelings of loneliness and isolation, stay mentally sharp, and improve your overall sense of well-being.

Overall, joining a senior center or club is a great way to stay active, socialize with others, and enhance your overall quality of life as you age. Whether you enjoy playing games, engaging in discussions, or learning new skills, there is sure to be a senior center or club that fits your interests and needs. So why wait? Joining a senior center or club today could be the beginning of a whole new chapter in your life as a senior citizen.

Volunteer Opportunities

Are you a senior citizen looking for ways to give back to your community and make a difference in the world? One of the best ways to do this is by volunteering your time and skills to help others in need. There are countless volunteer opportunities available for seniors, ranging from working with children and animals to assisting with environmental conservation projects. In this subchapter, we will explore some of the many ways in which you can get involved and make a positive impact through volunteering.

Volunteering is not only a great way to give back, but it also offers numerous benefits for seniors. Research has shown that volunteering can help improve mental and physical health, increase social connections, and provide a sense of purpose and fulfillment. By volunteering, you can stay active and engaged in your community, while also making a meaningful contribution to those in need. Whether you have a few hours a week or just a few minutes a day to spare, there are volunteer opportunities available to fit your schedule and interests.

One popular option for seniors looking to volunteer is working with children and youth. Many organizations, such as schools, daycares, and after-school programs, are in need of volunteers to help mentor, tutor, and support young people. By sharing your knowledge and life experiences with the next generation, you can make a lasting impact on their lives and help shape the future of your community. Whether you enjoy reading stories to children, helping with homework, or coaching sports teams, there are countless ways to get involved and make a difference in the lives of young people.

Another rewarding volunteer opportunity for seniors is working with animals. Animal shelters, rescue organizations, and wildlife sanctuaries are always in need of volunteers to help care for animals, socialize them, and assist with adoption events. By volunteering with animals, you can help provide much-needed love and attention to furry friends in need, while also getting the chance to spend time outdoors and stay active. Whether you have a passion for dogs, cats, horses, or wildlife, there are volunteer opportunities available to suit your interests and abilities.

In addition to working with children and animals, there are numerous other volunteer opportunities available for seniors, including assisting with environmental conservation projects, supporting local charities and nonprofits, and helping with community events and festivals. No matter what your interests and skills may be, there is sure to be a volunteer opportunity that aligns with your passions and values. By getting involved and giving back to your community, you can make a positive impact, stay active and engaged, and enjoy the many benefits that volunteering has to offer. So why not explore the volunteer opportunities available in your area and start making a difference today?

Planning Social Outings

Planning social outings can be a great way for senior citizens to stay active and engaged in their communities. It is important to consider factors such as transportation, accessibility, and interests when organizing these activities. By taking the time to plan ahead, seniors can ensure that they have enjoyable and fulfilling experiences with their friends and loved ones.

When planning a social outing, it is important to consider transportation options. Whether it be arranging for a ride with a friend or family member, utilizing public transportation, or hiring a car service, seniors should make sure they have a reliable way to get to and from their destination. It is also helpful to research parking options and any potential mobility issues that may arise at the location.

Accessibility is another key factor to consider when planning social outings. Seniors should make sure that the venue or activity is easily accessible for individuals with mobility challenges. This may involve checking for ramps, elevators, and designated parking spaces for those with disabilities. By choosing accessible venues, seniors can ensure that everyone can participate in the outing comfortably and safely.

When selecting activities for social outings, seniors should consider their interests and preferences. Whether it be attending a concert, visiting a museum, or simply going out for a meal with friends, it is important to choose activities that will be enjoyable and engaging for everyone involved. Seniors should also take into account any dietary restrictions or physical limitations that may impact their ability to participate in certain activities.

By planning social outings in advance and considering factors such as transportation, accessibility, and interests, seniors can ensure that they have rewarding and fulfilling experiences with their friends and loved ones. These outings provide opportunities for socialization, mental stimulation, and physical activity, all of which are important for maintaining overall health and well-being in the senior years. So go ahead and start planning your next social outing today!

Chapter 9: End of Life Planning

Discussing End-of-Life Wishes with Family

Discussing end-of-life wishes with family is a crucial and sensitive topic that all senior citizens should consider. It is important to have these conversations in order to ensure that your wishes are known and respected. By discussing your end-of-life wishes with your family, you can alleviate any potential stress or confusion that may arise in the future.

One of the first steps in discussing end-of-life wishes with family is to initiate the conversation. This may be a difficult and emotional discussion to have, but it is important to address the topic openly and honestly. Choose a time when everyone is calm and relaxed, and be sure to express your thoughts and feelings clearly.

Another important aspect of discussing end-of-life wishes with family is to be specific about your preferences. Consider creating an advance directive or living will that outlines your wishes for medical treatment, end-of-life care, and funeral arrangements. This document can serve as a guide for your family members and healthcare providers in the event that you are unable to communicate your wishes.

It is also important to involve your family members in the decision-making process. Listen to their concerns and opinions, and be open to their input. By involving your loved ones in the discussion, you can ensure that everyone is on the same page and that your wishes are understood and respected.

In conclusion, discussing end-of-life wishes with family is a difficult but necessary conversation for all senior citizens to have. By initiating the discussion, being specific about your preferences, and involving your family members in the decision-making process, you can ensure that your wishes are known and respected. Remember that having these conversations can provide peace of mind for both you and your loved ones in the future.

Funeral and Burial Planning

Funeral and burial planning is an important aspect of preparing for the end of life. It is a topic that many senior citizens may find difficult to discuss, but it is essential to ensure that your wishes are carried out and your loved ones are not burdened with making difficult decisions during a time of grief.

When it comes to funeral planning, there are several key decisions that need to be made. First and foremost, you will need to decide whether you want to be buried or cremated. This decision will impact the type of funeral service you have, as well as the costs involved. It is important to discuss your wishes with your loved ones so that they are aware of your preferences.

In addition to deciding on burial or cremation, you will also need to consider other aspects of your funeral service, such as the location, date, and type of service. Some senior citizens may choose to pre-plan their funeral service, which can help alleviate the stress and burden on their loved ones after they pass away. Pre-planning allows you to make all the necessary arrangements in advance, ensuring that your wishes are carried out exactly as you want.

When it comes to burial planning, there are also important decisions to be made. You will need to choose a burial plot, select a casket or urn, and decide on any additional services or memorials that you would like. It is important to consider these decisions carefully and discuss them with your loved ones to ensure that your wishes are respected.

Overall, funeral and burial planning are important aspects of preparing for the end of life. By taking the time to make these decisions in advance, you can ensure that your wishes are carried out and your loved ones are not burdened with making difficult decisions during a time of grief. Planning ahead can provide peace of mind for both you and your family, allowing you to focus on enjoying your remaining time together.

Hospice Care Options

When facing a terminal illness or end-of-life care, hospice care can provide comfort and support for both the patient and their loved ones. Hospice care focuses on quality of life and aims to manage pain and symptoms while providing emotional and spiritual support. There are several options available for seniors who are considering hospice care, and it's important to understand what each option entails.

One option for hospice care is in-home care, where a team of healthcare professionals come to the patient's home to provide care and support. This option allows the patient to remain in the comfort of their own home while receiving the necessary medical attention. In-home hospice care can also provide respite for family caregivers and help them navigate the challenges of caring for a loved one with a terminal illness.

Another option for hospice care is a hospice facility, where patients can receive around-the-clock care in a specialized facility. Hospice facilities are equipped to provide medical, emotional, and spiritual support to patients and their families. These facilities often have a team of healthcare professionals, including doctors, nurses, social workers, and spiritual counselors, who work together to provide comprehensive care for the patient.

For seniors who prefer a more holistic approach to hospice care, there are alternative options such as integrative hospice care. This type of care combines traditional medical treatments with complementary therapies such as massage, acupuncture, and music therapy. Integrative hospice care aims to address the physical, emotional, and spiritual needs of the patient, providing a more well-rounded approach to end-of-life care.

It's important for seniors and their families to explore their options and choose the hospice care option that best suits their needs and preferences. By understanding the different types of hospice care available, seniors can make informed decisions about their end-of-life care and ensure that they receive the support and comfort they need during this challenging time. No matter which option they choose, hospice care can provide peace of mind and compassionate care for seniors and their loved ones.

Chapter 10: Resources and Support Networks

Finding Local Senior Services

As we age, it becomes increasingly important to have access to local senior services that can help us navigate the challenges of getting older. Whether you need assistance with medical care, transportation, or social activities, there are a variety of resources available to help make your life easier and more enjoyable. In this chapter, we will explore some of the best ways to find local senior services in your area.

One of the best ways to find local senior services is to contact your local Area Agency on Aging. These agencies are dedicated to helping older adults access the services they need to live independently and with dignity. They can provide information on a wide range of services, including home care, transportation, meal delivery, and more. By reaching out to your local Area Agency on Aging, you can get connected to the resources that will help you thrive in your golden years.

Another great way to find local senior services is to contact your city or county government. Many municipalities offer programs and services specifically designed for older adults, such as senior centers, transportation services, and wellness programs. By reaching out to your local government, you can learn about the services available in your area and how to access them.

In addition to government agencies, there are also many nonprofit organizations that provide valuable services to seniors. These organizations may offer everything from social activities to home repair services to financial assistance. By researching local nonprofits that specialize in senior services, you can find the support you need to live a happy and healthy life in your later years.

In conclusion, finding local senior services is essential for older adults who want to live independently and with dignity. By reaching out to your local Area Agency on Aging, city or county government, and nonprofit organizations, you can access the resources you need to thrive in your golden years. Don't hesitate to ask for help when you need it - there are plenty of services available to support you as you navigate the challenges of aging.

Support Groups for Seniors

Support groups for seniors can be a valuable resource for those looking to connect with others who are going through similar experiences. These groups provide a supportive and understanding environment where seniors can share their concerns, seek advice, and build meaningful relationships with others in their age group. Many support groups focus on specific topics such as chronic illness, grief, caregiving, or retirement, allowing seniors to find a group that best suits their needs.

Attending a support group can help seniors feel less isolated and more connected to their community. It can be comforting to know that others are going through similar challenges and that there is a place where they can discuss their feelings openly and without judgment. Support groups often provide a sense of camaraderie and can help seniors build a support network that they can rely on in times of need.

In addition to emotional support, support groups for seniors can also provide practical advice and resources. Many groups invite guest speakers to discuss topics such as healthy aging, financial planning, or navigating the healthcare system. This can help seniors stay informed and empowered to make decisions that are in their best interests. Support groups can also be a great way to learn about local resources and services that can help seniors live more independently and comfortably.

Joining a support group can also have a positive impact on seniors' mental and physical well-being. Studies have shown that seniors who participate in support groups have lower levels of stress, anxiety, and depression. Social interaction and a sense of belonging can improve overall mental health and can even lead to better physical health outcomes. By connecting with others in a support group, seniors can feel more motivated to stay active, eat well, and take care of their overall well-being.

Overall, support groups for seniors can be a valuable tool for promoting social connection, emotional support, and practical resources. Whether you are dealing with a specific issue or simply looking to connect with others in your age group, joining a support group can have many benefits. If you are interested in finding a support group in your area, consider reaching out to local community centers, senior centers, or healthcare providers for recommendations. Remember, you are not alone - there are others who are going through similar experiences and are ready to offer their support and understanding.

Accessing Government Assistance Programs

Accessing government assistance programs can be a valuable resource for senior citizens looking to make ends meet or receive additional support in their golden years. These programs are designed to provide financial assistance, healthcare services, and other forms of support to seniors who may be facing challenges in their daily lives. By understanding how to access these programs and what benefits they offer, seniors can ensure they are receiving the assistance they need to live a comfortable and fulfilling life.

One of the most common government assistance programs for seniors is Social Security. This program provides monthly payments to eligible seniors based on their work history and contributions to the Social Security system. Seniors can apply for Social Security benefits online, over the phone, or in person at their local Social

Security office. By understanding the eligibility requirements and application process for Social Security benefits, seniors can ensure they are receiving the financial support they are entitled to.

Another important government assistance program for seniors is Medicare. Medicare is a federal health insurance program that provides coverage for hospital stays, doctor visits, prescription drugs, and other healthcare services for seniors aged 65 and older. Seniors can enroll in Medicare during specific enrollment periods, and there are different parts of the program that cover different services. By understanding how Medicare works and what services it covers, seniors can ensure they are receiving the healthcare they need to stay healthy and active.

In addition to Social Security and Medicare, there are other government assistance programs available to seniors, such as Medicaid, Supplemental Security Income (SSI), and the Low-Income Energy Assistance Program (LIHEAP). These programs provide additional financial assistance, healthcare services, and support with utility bills for seniors who may be struggling to make ends meet. By exploring these programs and understanding how to apply for them, seniors can access the resources they need to improve their quality of life and maintain their independence.

Overall, accessing government assistance programs can be a valuable resource for seniors looking to receive financial assistance, healthcare services, and other forms of support in their golden years. By understanding the various programs available, how to apply for them, and what benefits they offer, seniors can ensure they are receiving the assistance they need to live a comfortable and fulfilling life. It is important for seniors to explore all available resources and take advantage of the support that is available to them through government assistance programs.